Introduction to Ayurveda

Introduction to Ayurveda

Siân Pritchard-Jones
and Bob Gibbons

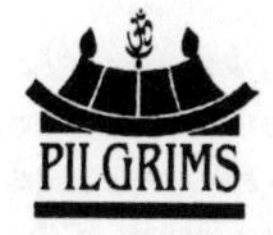

PILGRIMS PUBLISHING
◆ Varanasi ◆

Introduction to Ayurveda

Siân Pritchard-Jones and Bob Gibbons

Published by:
PILGRIMS PUBLISHING

An imprint of:
PILGRIMS BOOK HOUSE
(Distributors in India)
B 27/98 A-8, Nawabganj Road
Durga Kund, Varanasi-221010, India
Tel: 91-542- 2314060,
Fax: 91-542- 2312456
E-mail: pilgrims@satyam.net.in
Website: www.pilgrimsbooks.com

Layout and Cover design by Asha

ISBN: 81-7769-624-6

Printed in India at Pilgrim Press Pvt. Ltd. Lalpur Varanasi

Contents

Introduction

This concise book has been devised by Pilgrims Publications as an introduction to Ayurveda, produced in an easy-to-understand format. It gives a brief insight into the wide-ranging subject of Ayurveda. It is in no way a complete analysis of the subject. It is not concerned with the minute detail, or the complex and often confusing diagnosis and treatment of specific diseases that Ayurveda involves. It seeks to unravel some of the more basic ideas of Ayurveda and to delve into the more general topics within the subject. We leave it to students to refer to more specific books about the subject. Some are mentioned in the bibliography at the back of this book.

This book is a teaser for further exploration.

What is Ayurveda?

Ayurveda is the science of life. The word comes from the Sanskrit terms *ayus* meaning "life", and *veda* meaning "wisdom" or "science". It dates back over three thousand years ago, and indeed, some of these ancient textbooks are still in use today. There are four basic scriptures that evolved to become known as the Vedas. They have since developed to become the basic building blocks of Indian Philosophy.

History and Ayurveda

Ayurveda is older than time; no one is sure when it began. What is traditionally believed that in the India of three thousand or so years ago, fifty-two wise old men left their villages and went to the Himalayas, where they hoped to learn how to eradicate disease and sickness from the world of man. They were known as the *Rishis*. As they meditated together, they acquired the knowledge which is known today as Ayurveda. It was then written down and believed to be divinely inspired.

When the texts were written, disease was considered to be an evil visitation, which prevented man from achieving his goals on earth. A body suffering from disease would mean a spirit constrained by its earthly body, and unable to soar. To free someone from this would be to enable them to follow a truly spiritual path to enlightenment, liberated from the constraints of the physical body. One could only achieve enlightenment if one enjoyed both physical and mental well being.

Although started by Hindus, the knowledge of Ayurveda was later added to by Buddha, who died in 483 BC. Buddhism teaches that the mind can be enriched by correct thinking and that one should follow the middle way in order to survive the long journey through life. Following Buddha's teachings, more and more monks practised Ayurvedic medicine, and in Emperor Ashoka's time (272 – 231 BC) many Ayurvedic hospitals and Buddhist monasteries were established.

Despite the fact that around three-quarters of all Indians use Ayurveda, it was in danger of dying out in the early twentieth century, because it was considered old-fashioned and out-dated. But in 1921 Mahatma Gandhi opened the first college for Ayurvedic medicine in Delhi, and others opened soon after. In 1980 the Indian Congress credited Ayurvedic medicine with the same status as western medicine, and since then many more institutions have been established to teach Ayurveda, giving it the respect and finance it deserves.

Indian Philosophy and Ayurveda

All the different branches of Indian traditions and beliefs were inspired by the four Vedas. Although not set out in written form until much later, these wise scriptures now form the basis of all the life sciences found today. Whether one studies Yoga, Tantra, the Kama Sutra, Vaastu or Ayurveda, all have a common thread that bind the philosophies, practices, rituals and knowledge of each together within the Vedic ideals.

So what is this common thread?

It is in essence the idea that all and everything in the cosmos, the universe is inter- linked as one. Every object, living person, spirit, energy is connected and cannot be separated from the whole being. An action in one place of an object, atom, living being, creature, spirit is bound to cause an effect somewhere within the whole. For all ideas and actions a holistic approach is necessary. If we are to find the most harmonious path of life, we need to consider the energies of each and every object, living being and spiritual force.

On the human level, this means that any illness or disease must be considered within the framework of not only the body, but also all manner of external factors in which that body exists, including the infinity of space. It is only by first understanding that we must look at the infinite parameters of the whole that we can progress forward in expanding our knowledge of the practice of Ayurveda. Ayurveda is the practice of using these ideas of the whole in the search for a medical cure, in the same way that Vaastu, for example, is used to design a building. Both require the correct interpretation and analysis of the task, in relation to how that treatment or the siting of a new structure will react on the whole, in relation to the physical aspects, the spiritual aspects and the energy life forces within the cosmos.

Fundamental Concepts of Ayurveda

One of the ancient treatises or texts on Ayurveda, the Charak Samhita, states that health is said to exist in a body when the following conditions are present: —

a) All the three **doshas** are in balance
b) All the seven **dhatus** are working properly
c) The three **malas**, waste products, are produced and eliminated normally and in normal quantities
d) The **srotas**, channels, of the body are uninterrupted
e) The **agni**, digestive fire, is alight and the appetite is good
f) The five senses are functioning normally
g) Body, mind and consciousness are working in harmony.

We will now go on to explain many of these terms, an understanding of which is essential to a comprehension of Ayurveda.

Antimatter

What is life? A body, when dead, still consists of the same physical matter as when it was alive; skin, bone, blood and other tissues. Indeed, it has been noted that the hair and nails continue to grow even after death. Therefore even growth is not necessarily a sign of life.

So what is it that makes us alive? Consciousness, the sign of antimatter. Previously it was thought that the atom was the smallest entity that could exist, but it is now known that it can be broken down much further than that. Nuclear physicists likewise acknowledge that on both the atomic and sub-atomic level, antimatter is the driving force.

Antimatter, the soul, consciousness, is also known as **purusha**.

Prana

What is **prana**? Prana is the life force, the Sanskrit term meaning "Absolute Energy". It is important that we understand prana as the principle of energy exhibited in all living things. It is this which distinguishes them from lifeless things.

It is in all forms of matter, and yet it is not matter. It is in the air, but it is neither the air nor one of its constituents. We breathe it in with the air, and if the air did not contain it we would die. It is taken up by the system along with the oxygen, and yet is not the oxygen.

In the same way that the oxygen in the air is used by the blood and circulatory system, so is the prana used by the nervous system. Prana is carried to all parts of the nervous system, adding strength and vitality. By thinking of prana as the active principle of what we call "vitality," we can form a much clearer idea of what an important part it plays in our lives.

In order to cultivate and stimulate it, we must breathe in a correct and nourishing manner. To breathe is to live; without breath there is no life. We must allow this energy to flow freely throughout our bodies. Poor posture and bad thoughts, which make us fell angry and resentful, will block the flow of prana, making it impossible for our bodies to function harmoniously. When channelled effectively, prana enhances our wellbeing, creativity and development of the senses, bringing greater understanding. It is therefore important to cultivate this force when seeking to regenerate the body.

Prana is found in its freest state in the atmospheric air. Fresh air is full of it. Although the concept is not fully understood by Western doctors, they do recognise that the air in certain places possesses a greater amount of "something", and sick people are sent to these places in the hope of improving their state of health.

Past Lives and Reincarnation in Ayurveda

Reincarnation is a fundamental tenet of Ayurveda. The world appears to be a cruel, anarchic and unfair place where people suffer for no apparent reason, especially children. But if we believe in reincarnation, we can see that everything that happens is a result of something that happened long before; there is order in everything. Ayurveda believes that we each bring memories from our past lives, inheritance from our parents as well as our dosha influences. A factor which connects the different stages in our lives, while maintaining our individual identity, is called **smirti**. This is equivalent to memory, but it permeates every cell of our body.

The Five Elements

Panch Maha Bhutas (five great forces)

At the heart of Ayurvedic science lies the concept of the five elements. The *rishis* perceived intuitively that consciousness was energy manifested into the five basic principles of ether, air, fire, water and earth.

These five basic principles exist in all matter. For example, solid ice is a manifestation of the earth principle. From the latent heat within, the fire principle, it turns to water, with more heat (fire) it turns to steam (air), and eventually disappears into the ether. The five elements are related to the five senses as follows: —

Ether	—	*Hearing*
Air	—	*Touch*
Fire	—	*Sight*
Water	—	*Taste*
Earth	—	*Smell*

Ether is the medium through which sound is transmitted, so this is related to hearing. The ear is the organ of hearing and expresses itself through the mouth, the organ of speech, which creates meaningful sound.

Air is related to touch — the skin is the sensory organ of touch and the hand the main action organ. The fingertips are especially sensitive to touch, and thus the hand is used for giving, receiving and holding.

Fire (*Agni*) giving light, heat and colour, is related to sight. The organ of sight is the eye, and this is related to the feet, because sight gives direction to our walking.

Water is related to taste; for without water the tongue cannot taste. The tongue is related in function to the genitals. Ayurveda considers the genitals to be the lower tongue, while that in the mouth is the upper tongue. He or she who controls the upper tongue also controls the lower tongue.

Earth is related to smell. The nose, the organ of smell, is related to the anus, demonstrated by the fact that a person who has constipation is likely to have bad breath and a reduced sense of smell.

Although the human body consists mainly of water and earth, the other elements also exist within it. For example, all the hollow spaces, such as the throat, trachea, oesophagus, sinuses and ear canals consist of the element ether. The air in the lungs, vessels and pores within the bones is clearly air, and the digestive tract is a kind of fire.

Three Bio-Energies — Doshas

The human body is made up of a combination of three fundamental elements, known as the three doshas; Vata, Pitta, and Kapha. Only living matter has doshas. There is no exact equivalent in the English language; the closest translation is "fault", or "that which causes things to decay". Each and every one of us is a unique individual, with a different combination of the three doshas. Hence we may say that a person is predominantly Vata or Pitta, for example.

The doshas regulate the physical, physiological and psychological functions of the living organism. For good health, it is important that all three doshas are balanced. If any of these doshas is out of equilibrium, either too high or too low, disease will occur.—

Vata—is in charge of all motion in the body, and it governs most nervous functions.

Pitta—governs enzymes and hormones, all forms of transformation and bio-chemical changes. It is also responsible for digestion of food and reaction to sensory data received by the brain, for example temperature, hunger, thirst, sight etc.

Kapha—regulates the other two doshas, nourishing and preserving the human body. It is a stabilising influence, responsible for the solidity of the body, sexual power and reproduction, strength, patience etc.

Although existing throughout the whole body, each dosha is prominent in certain parts of the body:—

Vata—below the navel; bladder, intestines, pelvic region, thighs, legs, bones.

Pitta—between the navel and chest; sweat, lymph, blood, stomach. Liver, spleen, gall bladder, stomach, duodenum, pancreas.

Kapha—upper part; thorax, head, neck, joints, upper portions of stomach, fatty tissues, sinuses, nostrils, throat, bronchi, lungs.

Vata—controls all movement in the body, and because of this it is considered to be the most influential dosha. It is composed of Air and Space. It controls breathing and elimination, both vitally important functions without which we cannot live. It controls the empty spaces within a body, for example the sinuses, lungs and inner ear as well as the abdominal cavity and the nervous system. It controls the nervous system, cell division and recreation, as well as the heart, which causes blood to flow throughout the body.

A person with predominant Vata is likely to be light in weight and with a creative mind. They may also be flippant in attitude or unreliable. Usually thin and athletic, but not very muscly, their voice may be thin and high. They will probably have dry skin and a very rapid metabolism, not putting on weight easily. Quick to learn, they are equally quick to forget and prone to anxiety.

Too much vata can cause the whole body to be dehydrated, with premature ageing and slow healing of wounds. It can also cause a darker complexion, a hacking cough and dark urine and faeces. Insufficient vata can cause sluggishness and bad circulation.

They prefer sweet, sour and salty foods and hot drinks.

Pitta—energy is composed of Fire and Water. It is sited mainly in the stomach, and governs the production and retention of body heat, digestion, metabolism and intelligence.

Pitta people generally tend to the middle ground. They have lustrous skin, possibly with moles or freckles, and go grey or bald early. With a sharp appetite, their metabolism is strong. They tend to have warm bodies, and perspire freely. Moderately well off, they are good organisers and decision-makers, as well as being open to new ideas. Highly intelligent, they are often good speakers but can tend to be judgmental and jealous.

Someone with excessive pitta is likely to have an abnormally high body temperature possibly caused by infection or inflammation, and to be thirsty, sweaty and tired. The skin and eyes may appear yellowish.

They prefer sweet, bitter and astringent food and cold drinks.

Kapha—energy is composed of Water and Earth. It controls water-based functions, such as lubrication of joints, and governs strength and mass, as well as maintaining the immune system.

Kapha people tent to have well built bodies and can be overweight. Their veins and bone structure are not prominent because of the fatty layers. The skin is lustrous, as is the hair, and the eyes tend to be full and bright. They have good stamina levels, moving slowly but definitely. Their memories are good, though they are slower to learn in the first place. Being generally healthy and happy, they are also tolerant and forgiving; when they earn money they are good at keeping it and are not spendthrifts.

Someone with excessive kapha is likely to be overweight, with loose joints and impotence. Digestion may be slow and they may suffer heartburn.

They prefer pungent, bitter and astringent foods.

Prakruti—means the individual constitution, which is decided in the womb. Each person's prakruti depends on the combination of the three doshas, and will be different for each and every one of us. This is the reason why Ayurveda looks at the whole patient when identifying a way to treat the disease. Each dosha has an effect on the mental, anatomical and physiological activities of an individual.

Mental Constitution

As well as the physical constitutional factors described above, the doshas, there are also three types of mental constitution, known as the three *gunas*. These are **sattva**, **rajas** and **tamas**.

People with a **Sattva** constitution are generally very loving, kind, understanding, pure and compassionate. They usually enjoy good health, perhaps because of a lack of stress in their lives. Most of them believe in God, and they are often very holy. It is much easier for them to achieve self-realisation than the other two types.

A **Rajas** constitution implies great sensuality and an extrovert personality. These people are prosperous, but can tend to be aggressive. They enjoy movement and are often wealthy businessmen or involved in politics.

Tamas people are ignorant, lazy, dull and egotistical. They show no respect to others and are often the cause of others' undoing. With their selfish attitudes, they find it almost impossible to achieve self-realisation.

These mental energies, which are responsible for our behavioural patterns, can be improved markedly through yoga. An Ayurvédic doctor can help by prescribing changes in lifestyle and diet as well as other treatments.

Six Tastes (Shad Rasa)

With our sense of taste, we can identify six principle varieties as follows:—

Sweet	earth and water
Sour	earth and fire
Salty	water and fire
Bitter	air and ether
Pungent	air and fire
Astringent	air and earth

It is important to stimulate all the taste buds; remember the phrase "use it or lose it". A meal should ideally consist of something with each of the six flavours, in order that all the taste buds will be activated.

In addition, the six tastes each have different properties, some of which are listed below:—

Sweet e.g. fruit, liquorice; soothing, laxative, relieves thirst, supports immune system.

Sour e.g. lemon, cider vinegar, yoghurt; calms stomach, relieves thirst.

Salty e.g. seaweed; softening, mildly sedative, stimulates digestion, laxative.

Bitter e.g. rhubarb, fenugreek; antitoxic and germicidal, soothes itching and burning.

Pungent e.g. ginger, cayenne, garlic; causes sweating, promotes digestion and metabolism, reduces nausea.

Astringent e.g. unripe banana, turmeric; stops bleeding, heals wounds, prevents diarrhoea.

Seven Tissues (Sapta Dhatus)

The human body is made up of basically seven different types of tissue. Like the doshas, these are made of one or more of the five elements, but unlike the doshas, they can be seen with the naked eye. In Sanskrit they are known as the *sapta dhatus*.

The first of these is plasma *(Rasa dhatu)*. This is the basis of the formation of blood *(Rakta dhatu)*, which flows through muscles *(Mamsa dhatu)*. Then follow *fatty tissue (Meda dhatu)*, bone *(Asthi dhatu)*, marrow and nerve tissue *(Majja dhatu)* and finally reproductive tissue *(Shukra dhatu)*. Each of these tissues is derived from the preceding one; the last has the greatest potential, that of creating new life.

Rasa Dhatu

When we take in food the metabolic processes begin. Initially the digestive juices act, and then after this the *agni* or fire of the stomach begins to convert the food which becomes nutrients for the body. The plasma or Rasa Dhatu is the means of transport of these nutrients. Healthy Rasa is seen as rich skin, vitality, joy and a focussed manner. When Rasa is poor there is aching, heaviness and nausea, which are features of increased kapha.

Rakta Dhatu

The Rakta Dhatu are the elements of the blood, the red and white cells, the platelets which hold the life-giving fire, the oxygen in particular. Oxygen is needed for nourishment of the tissues and the mind. Healthy Rakta gives fullness and richness to lips, tongue, nails, hands and feet. It gives enthusiasm, feeling and awareness. When Rakta is excessive, there is inflammation.

Mamsa Dhatu

The Mamsa Dhatu maintains the physical strength of the body and protects the internal organs. It has earth as its main element and corresponds to the muscular tissues. The health of the Mamsa can be seen in the muscles of the body, including those around the face and head. Strength, stability and a sense of belonging come with a healthy Mamsa. Too much Mamsa will bring fat, lethargy and sloth. Too little can bring wasting, weakness and fear.

Meda Dhatu

The Meda Dhatu corresponds to fatty substances and its elements are water and earth. It is the lubricant of the body and comes from the Mamsa. Flexibility comes with good Meda, and with that a sense of compassion, honesty and wellbeing. Increased Meda causes fat to accumulate around the midriff, with subsequent respiratory problems. A lowering of Meda causes numbness, cracking in joints and atrophy.

Asthi Dhatu

The Asthi Dhatu is reflected in bone tissue, and is of the elements earth and air. Strong bones and joints are a reflection of healthy Asthi, as well as an enjoyment of life, optimism and trustworthiness.

Too much Asthi will result in prominent teeth, bony prominences of joints and skull. Too little can mean stiff joints, brittle nails and thin hair.

Majja Dhatu

Majja Dhatu represents bone marrow. Its principal element is water. Healthy Majja will result in a good voice and a supple body, which enjoys dance and has a good immune system. Too much Majja can lead to chronic pain and infection in the bones, as well as chronic fatigue. Too little can result in joint pain, fragility of bones and frequent dizziness.

Shukra Dhatu

This dhatu is nourished by all the others. It represents the sexual and reproductive tissues of the male and female; the sperm and the ovum. Its principal element is water. Healthy Shukra will result in a healthy sexual appetite for the opposite sex, personal charisma and fertility, as well as boundless energy for spiritual and physical activities. Too much Shukra can result in an abnormally high sexual desire, especially in men. Women may experience heavier and more frequent periods, and perhaps lactation even when not nursing a child. Too little can result in impotence in men and irregular periods in women as well as chronic fatigue.

Just as one or two of the doshas may predominate in any one individual, so may the dhatus. In fact, when the doshas are in balance they also are regarded as dhatus. It is only when then are disturbed that they are considered to be doshas, i.e. "faults".

Waste Products (*Mala*)

These are three; faeces (*purisha*), urine (*mutra*) and sweat (*sveda*).

Unless we are able to excrete these waste products, illness will result.

Faeces (*Purisha*)

Every day approximately 8 – 9 litres of fluid is absorbed by the digestive tract. About 2 litres comes from drinking and eating; the rest comes from saliva and other internal secretions. Out of all this fluid, only 1 litre or so reaches the colon; the rest is absorbed back into the body. The function of the colon is to convert this waste fluid into a solid mass that can be excreted as faeces. The important processes which occur are the reabsorption of the remaining fluid and electrolytes into the body, the peristaltic movements which push the faeces further down the colon and help to dry it out, and finally defecation.

The principal element in purisha is earth. The most important dosha is vata, but all the doshas play their part in elimination. If there is any imbalance in the three doshas, uncomfortable symptoms will manifest in the process of elimination of the faeces. Too much faeces production will result in a heavy, full abdomen and lower bowel, flatulence and gurgling. Too little can produce symptoms of bloating with upper abdominal pain. Abnormal bowel function can also result in other diseases not directly connected with the intestinal tract, such as rheumatoid arthritis, osteoarthritis, bronchitis, asthma, sciatica, lower back pain, dysmenorrhea, headaches etc. It can also cause metabolic disorders such as low potassium and calcium levels etc.

Urine (*Mutra*)

The urinary system removes nitrogenous wastes from the body. It helps to regulate fluid balance, affecting the blood pressure and production of red blood cells. The formation of urine begins in the colon, where large amounts of fluid are transported to the kidneys. More processing takes place here, then the urine is transferred to the bladder before final elimination. The main element of urine is water, but it also includes fire.

Too much urine production can result in bladder and kidney infections. Too little can result in kidney stones, thirst and abdominal pain.

Sweat (*Sveda*)

Sweat originates in the fatty tissues. It helps to maintain a correct body temperature, as well as regulating the electrolyte balance in the body and the bacteria on the surface of the skin. Too much sweat can result in skin infections such as ringworm. It can also cause itching, bad odours and sometimes chilling of the body. Too little can cause overheating, burning sensations and dry skin.

Other waste products are nails, hair, earwax and dead skin cells. However, since they do not cause disease, they are not of interest in our understanding of Ayurveda.

Channels (*Srotas*)

Channels within the body, along which substances are transported, are called *srotas*. These channels allow nutrients to enter the body, and waste products to be excreted from the body, as well as providing a means for blood to flow and send nutrients throughout the tissues.

The largest of these is the gastro-intestinal tract. Others include the oesophagus, the urinary system, plus of course the arteries, innumerable veins and capillaries through which the blood flows to every part of the body, and the lungs and bronchi which provide the blood with fresh oxygen and prana.

Other channels do not exist in a physical sense; no anatomy student will find them when dissecting a human body. Nevertheless, they are very similar to the meridian in Chinese medicine.

A blockage in any of these channels can have serious, if not fatal, consequences and it is therefore essential to keep them free of obstruction. Several factors may result in blocked *srotas*: physical injury, disturbed doshas or a mental blow such as bereavement. Often a Western patient may not know they have a blocked *srota* until symptoms of a fully-fledged disease have presented. It is the aim of Ayurveda to make sure that the *srotas* do not become blocked in the first place and that disease cannot ensue.

Malfunctions of the *srotas* leading to illness can be classified in four ways: excessive circulation, insufficient circulation, blocked circulation and damage to a channel. Excessive circulation can cause over development of an organ, while insufficient can lead to failure to excrete waste products adequately. A blocked channel can result in a build-up of waste products or undigested food, leading to atrophy of the organ or surrounding tissues. Damage to a channel, for example during an accident, can result in blockage, and waste products may try to find a new way round the obstacle, coming into contact with incompatible tissues and thereby causing further problems.

In one of the ancient texts, Susruta describes nine channels, which physically exist and have openings to the outside of the body:

Eyes, ears, nose, mouth, anus and urethra for both sexes, and for women:

Two breast nipples (producing milk) and the vagina.

Of course, both sexes also have innumerable pores in the skin which allow sweat to escape; these are very minor channels but still perform an essential role.

Caraka, another ancient text, describes thirteen different channels, and the products which move through them:

Prana Vaha Srota	—	prana
Anna Vaha Srota	—	food
Udaka Vaha Srota	—	serum and lymph, protein-containing fluids
Rasa Vaha Srota	—	plasma
Rakta Vaha Srota	—	blood
Mamsa Vaha Srota	—	muscle fibre
Medo Vaha Srota	—	fatty tissue

Ashti Vaha Srota	—	bone tissue
Majja Vaha Srota	—	cerebrospinal fluids and bone marrow
Shukra Vaha Srota	—	reproductive tissues including semen and ovaries
Sveda Vaha Srota	—	sweat
Purisha Vaha Srota	—	stool
Mutra Vaha Srota	—	urine

Eight Branches or Specialities of Ayurveda

The main branches of Ayurvedic medicine are listed below. However, nowadays surgery is normally left to Western medicine, as it is conceded that those methods are generally superior. Ayurveda is particularly effective when dealing with chronic illnesses for which conventional medicine has failed to find a cure, and mental problems.

General internal medicine
Surgery
Ear, Nose and Throat and ophthalmology
Pediatrics
Geriatrics
Sexology, aphrodisiacs
Toxicology
Psychiatry and Psychology

Disease

What is disease? At the risk of unnecessary repetition, we have said earlier that the body is considered to be healthy when:—

a) All the three *doshas* are in balance
b) All the seven *dhatus* are working properly
c) The three *malas*, waste products, are produced and eliminated normally and in normal quantities
d) The *srotas*, channels, of the body are uninterrupted
e) The *agni*, digestive fire, is alight and the appetite is good
f) The five senses are functioning normally
g) Body, mind and consciousness are working in harmony.

Therefore, any disturbance to any of the above will imply bad health or disease. Health is order;

disease is disorder. Where there is order, there is always the possibility of disorder. The human body is a complex organism and it must be carefully monitored to recognise and control symptoms and causes of disease. Often we can tell that our body is not feeling quite right, even when there are no obvious symptoms to help identify any recognisable disease.

The internal functions of our bodies are constantly reacting to the external functions and environment. When we cannot change the external environment, Ayurveda shows us how to change the internal environment to bring it into balance with the external. With balance comes order and with order comes health. A balance of the above elements is responsible for our immune system and natural resistance to disease.

When our bodies are healthy and well balanced, our resistance to disease is improved and we are less likely to fall ill, even when confronted by infections and contagious diseases. It is imbalances of the body and mind that are largely responsible for both physical and psychological pain and suffering.

Classification of disease

Ayurveda classifies disease according to its origin; psychological, spiritual or physical. It is also classified according to where it is, for example in the lungs, legs or wherever. Disease may occur in one place but the symptoms may manifest in another. Diseases are also classified according to the cause and the bodily dosha.

Dosha and disease

Certain dosha types will be more prone to certain diseases. For example, kapha people are more prone to kapha diseases, which are tonsillitis, bronchitis, sinusitis and lung congestion. Pitta people are more prone to diseases of the abdomen such as gallbladder problems, liver disorders, peptic ulcers and gastritis, as well as skin diseases. Vata people are more susceptible to lower back pain, wind, arthritis and sciatica.

The imbalance causing the disease may first begin in the mind. For example, repressed fear will aggravate vata, repressed anger will aggravate pitta and repressed greed will aggravate kapha. But the opposite is also true; too much pitta energy in the body will cause anger to develop and so on. Imbalances that first manifest on one level can transfer to the other level; mental disorders can have physical effects and vice versa. We all know how pain can make us irritable and upset, and conversely how grief can make us ill.

There is a direct connection between diet, lifestyle, the environment and health disorders. By modifying our diet and lifestyle, even if we are unable to change our environment, we can still have a significant impact on our state of health.

Disturbances of the tridosha create toxins (*ama*), which then circulate throughout the body in the bloodstream. These will tend to stop in any point of weakness and cause disease there.

Diagnosis

In the West, diagnosis normally occurs after a disease has manifested, and the patient has gone to the doctor with a presentable case. But in Ayurveda, the doctor tries to identify the disease before it has happened, i.e. it can be used as a form of preventative medicine. This concept implies a regular monitoring of the interactions between order and disorder in the body. The symptoms of disease are always related to disturbances in the balance of the three doshas, and once this has been established, treatment can begin.

Ayurveda teaches the precise methods for determining the disease process before any outward signs are visible. By carefully monitoring your own body, you can determine what disease process is going on before it develops into an illness. Early diagnosis can often help to prevent a disease from developing, or at the very least to reduce its impact. The human body is a living book and, to understand it, it must be read daily.

Pulse

The pulse is normally checked at the wrist (radial pulse), but it can be checked at various other points of the body.

1) temporal artery, just above the temple on the side of the head
2) carotid artery, on the side of the neck above the collarbone
3) brachial artery, on the inside of the arm above the elbow
4) radial artery on the wrist
5) femoral artery on the inside front of the leg where it joins the pelvis
6) posterior tibial artery on the foot behind the ankle
7) dorsalis pedis artery on top of the foot

The radial pulse should be felt with the first three fingers of the hand, with the index finger closest to the wrist. It can be different on both sides of the body, therefore both sides should be noted. It should not be taken after sex, exertion, massage, eating or bathing, as this will give an inaccurate reading.

By decreasing the pressure on each finger, one can sense the varying movements of the pulse and determine which is predominant.

The position of the index finger denotes the pulse of vata. If this pulse predominates, the index finger feels the throbbing of the pulse more strongly. This pulse feels like a snake, quick and slithery. 80 – 100 beats per minute.

The middle finger denotes the pulse of pitta. If this pulse is the strongest, it is active and jumpy like a frog. 70 – 80 beats per minute.

The ring finger denotes the pulse of kapha. If this pulse is the strongest, it is slow and resembles the floating of a swan. 60 – 70 beats per minute.

Tongue Diagnosis

The tongue can be used as a diagnostic tool by noting any discolouration or sensitivity. Different parts of the tongue correspond to different parts of the body, and by "reading" the tongue we can identify which part of the body is diseased. A whitish tongue is an indication of a kapha disturbance and an accumulation of mucus. Similarly, a reddish or yellowy-green tongue indicates a pitta problem, and a black tongue implies a vata disturbance. If the tongue is dehydrated, there is a reduction in the plasma (Rasa Dhatu), and a pale tongue indicates a low red blood cell count (Rakta Dhatu).

Look at your tongue in the mirror. This is a very important organ, both for speech and taste. The tongue must be moist to taste anything; a dry tongue has no sense of taste.

Look at the size, shape and coating of the tongue. If it is pale, anaemia is likely. If it is yellow, there may be an excess of bile in the gall bladder or a liver disease. If it is blue, there may be a heart defect (provided you have not been eating blueberries!)

Indentations of the teeth along the side of the tongue indicate poor intestinal absorption. If the tongue is coated, the position of the coating indicates the area of disturbance in the body; the back of the tongue represents the large intestine, the middle represents the stomach and small intestine.

A line down the middle of the tongue indicates emotions being stored in the vertebrae. If the line is crooked, it can mean backache in the corresponding part of the back, or it may mean a deformity in the spine.

Facial Diagnosis

By facial diagnosis, we mean that the skin of the face can give a lot of clues as to the state of health of the individual. Horizontal lines across the forehead are a sign of worry. A vertical line between the eyebrows, on the left or right respectively, can imply emotions/anger held in the spleen or liver respectively.

Puffy lower eyelids (water retention) can mean kidney malfunction.

Lip Diagnosis

Lips in particular can tell us a lot about a person's health. If they are dry, rough and thin, there is a vata disturbance. Pale lips indicate anaemia. Frequent attacks of herpes on the lips can indicate a pitta derangement. Kapha lips tend to be thick and oily. Brown spots on the lips can mean poor digestion and/or worms.

Nail Diagnosis

Ayurveda teaches that the nails are a waste product of the bones. By observing their shape and form we can learn a lot. For example, if they are dry and rough, and break easily, vata is predominant. If they are soft and pink, flexible and easily bent, pitta predominates. And if they are thick, strong and uniform, then kapha is dominant.

Longitudinal lines in the nails indicate malabsorption of food by the digestive system. Transverse lines indicate an chronic illness or bad nutrition.

Prominent and convex nails, known as club nails, indicate a delicate heart or lungs. A nail which is concave and will hold a drop of water indicates an iron deficiency, while white spots indicate a lack of zinc or calcium.

Pale nails are an indication of anaemia, and if they are very red there is likely to be an excess of red blood cells. Yellow nails are an indication of jaundice or liver problems, and blue nails indicate a weak heart.

Each finger and thumb correspond to an organ of the body. (Cf. reflexology and the feet.)

Eye Diagnosis

Changes in the eyes can point to malfunctioning bio-energies.

Dominant vata results in small dry eyes, deep-set and anxious, with excessive blinking showing a tendency to nervousness and fear. If the upper eyelid droops, it may indicate a sense of insecurity or lack of confidence.

With overactive kapha, the eyes are likely to be watery, whitish, shiny but not brilliant. But they will probably appear large and attractive.

Pitta dominance can present as red eyes, possibly with a discharge at the corners and. They have a tendency to be near-sighted. Because of the fire in a pitta body, the eyes are often sensitive to light.

Other Tests

Apart from all the diagnostic tests we have discussed here, Ayurveda also studies other parts of the body and performs other clinical tests to arrive at a correct diagnosis.

Treatment

All Ayurvedic treatments aim to balance the three bodily humours; Vata, Pitta and Kapha. Disease results when these three are out of balance.

According to Ayurvedic teaching, treatment cannot be effective if the body is not first cleansed and toxins eliminated. Symptomatic relief may be obtained, but the underlying cause of the disease will still be there and the disease is likely to recur, in the same or a different form.

There are basically two types of treatment – elimination of toxins and neutralisation of toxins. These can be applied on either the physical level, or the emotional / mental level.

Emotional

In our lives in the West, we are taught to control our emotions and not to show negative emotions in public. Anger, fear, jealousy, possessiveness and greed are bottled up inside us. But if these emotions are not allowed to pass through us, and are held within our bodies, they will manifest as health problems in various parts of the body. Ayurveda teaches us to release those emotions, to recognise them and let them go.

Physical

Before the body is ready for Ayurvedic drugs, it needs to be cleansed of all impurities. The *pancha karma* means the five methods of cleansing. Normally in the West we do not recommend vomiting, because of its association with bulimia. When it is recommended, it must be closely supervised by a doctor because of the other dangers of uncontrolled vomiting.

Pancha Karma

The five methods of cleansing are:—

vomiting, emesis, (*Vamana*)
purging with laxatives (*Virecana*)
medicated enemas (*Vasti*)

nasal medicine (*Nasya*)
blood purification (*Rakta Moksha*)

Emesis (vomiting) is said by some authors to be the most effective means of normalising kapha in the body. It is used mainly to combat kapha disorders such as indigestion, sinusitis, headaches, catarrh, asthma and chronic coughs. The patient's stomach is filled with a liquid combination of water, milk and sugar, plus a selected medication to initiate vomiting. There are 22 different medications that the doctor can choose from to initiate emesis. His choice will depend on whether it is only kapha which is disturbed, or whether pitta and vata also need to be normalised. While the patient is vomiting, the doctor will be close at hand, helping the patient by rubbing his back, sides, navel region and forehead. If the vomit contains any traces of blood, the process must be stopped at once. When vomiting stops, the patient should feel relieved. He should then rest and take a hot bath.

Purging (medically induced elimination of stool) is an ideal treatment for pitta-related illnesses. It is also used for kapha-pitta disorders, and kapha disorders which have become lodged in pitta locations. This treatment is mainly used for skin complaints, asthma, urine retention, constipation, headaches and other toxic conditions. It can be done at home, so long as it is supervised by a qualified Ayurvedic doctor. The patient's digestive capacity is first calculated and then laxatives are taken orally. After many eliminations – thirty is considered very successful, twenty moderately successful, and ten poor – the colon is considered cleansed.

Enemas are of two types, oily and herbal decoctions. They are also differentiated by the passage through which they are administered; some are rectal, some urethral and others vaginal. This treatment is considered by some to be the most important form of Pancha Karma treatment. It is used for vata-related diseases.

In general, oily enemas stay inside the patient for nine hours, though in special cases this may be increased to twenty-four. The amount of oil used is 80 – 240 ml. This treatment can be used for some time, as it strengthens the body and rejuvenates it.

On the contrary, enemas using herbal concoctions should not stay in the body for more than 45 minutes. These enemas are used after oil enemas, to prevent the intestine from drying out. Usually they have sour characteristics, but may also be made up of milk, honey and herbs. For constipation a mix of 120 ml of milk, 60 ml of caster oil, 20 ml of honey and 6 g of natural mineral salt is recommended. This first produces faeces, then bile, and finally mucous matter. After this treatment the patient should feel light and refreshed, not weak.

Nasal Medicine is the application of drops of oil, or powder, to the nose. This is a good method of administering medicine to the head. One method, which can be used every day and at any time of year, is to dip a finger into oil and use this to massage the inside of the nose with the fingertip. This provides protection against colds and prevents the mucous membranes from drying out. But if the mucous membranes are to be treated, oil therapy should not be used beforehand.

Phlebotomy is the process of bloodletting, to remove toxins from the body. Leeches are sometimes used for special purposes. Or a small amount of blood may be extracted from a vein, by cutting the skin in sterile conditions with a surgical instrument.

Once the body has been effectively cleansed, it is then ready for treatment, with massage, lifestyle modification, dietary changes, Ayurvedic medicines or surgery.

It is beyond the scope of this book to go further down this line; it is necessary to consult an Ayurvedic doctor to determine the actual treatment necessary. But we will continue now with a discussion of massage therapies.

Massage

Massage is a frequently used form of Ayurvedic treatment, using oils, the marma points and the chakras.

Marma Points

Throughout the body are 107 energy points, known as marma points. These stimulate some of the functions of the body and maintain a state of health, by keeping all the functions in balance. They cannot be measured by science – they are similar to the Chinese meridians in this respect. But there is evidence to show that whenever one of them gets blocked or malfunctions for whatever reason, the body will display signs of illness.

The marma points are generally found where two different systems meet, for example, where nerves meet blood vessels, bones meet tendons or ligaments meet joints. Energy is concentrated at these points, and if they suffer grave injury, serious illness can result. The three main marma centres are the heart, head and bladder. A violent injury to either of these sites can cause death.

The marma points may be used in massage to manipulate the bio-energies of vata, pitta and kapha.

Chakras

What are the chakras? In Sanskrit, chakra means wheel. There are six chakras within the body and a seventh outside the body, hovering just above the head. They are the locations of vital energy and life force. They are reality when projected by the mind as a visual image. There is some evidence from a scientific and medical perspective that these energy points do exist. The chakras are vital for the transmission of energy to raise awareness. They each have a symbolic colour. The seven chakras are located and described as follows:—

The first chakra is the **Muladhara**, which is the root chakra. This is the creative force of the universe and is located in the genital area. It is the centre for awakening and basic survival. It is connected to the nose and gives us the sense of smell. This base chakra is the point from which the *Kundalini* force rises up. The colour of this chakra is deep crimson; this is the earth chakra.

The second chakra is the **Svadisthana** and it is located in the belly below the navel. In this chakra we deal with the fertility and creativity of the mother goddess. Here is desire and sexual need. The life force is expressed as pain or pleasure from here. Taste is also represented here. The colour of this chakra is dark blue; this is the water chakra.

The third chakra is **Manipura**, located near the solar plexus. It is devoted to digestion. It is concerned with vitality, energy and power. It deals with assimilation of the forces. It has power over the ego and the mental body. This is usually the first chakra to be activated. The colour of this chakra is also dark blue; this is the chakra of fire.

The fourth chakra is **Anahata**. This is the heart chakra, devoted to love and passion, which is between the body and the consciousness. It is concerned with harmonisation and vibrations. It is connected with touch and the immune system. The colour of this chakra is deep red; it is the air chakra.

The fifth chakra is **Vissudha**, the throat chakra. It is concerned with sound, hearing, speech and breathing. Balance is paramount in connection with this chakra. The thyroid gland is of importance in this chakra. This chakra is connected to hearing. Its colour is smoky grey; this is the ether chakra.

The sixth chakra is **Ajna**. This is particularly important and resides on the forehead as the Third Eye. It connects the higher and lower mind life force centres. The pineal and pituitary glands are important here. This chakra gives rise to any psychic vision, allowing us to see things as they really are. The colour of this chakra is silvery white; it is the mind chakra.

The seventh and last chakra is **Sahasrana**. It is located above the head and is the seat of enlightenment. All other chakras are connected to this chakra. It is linked to the brain and its power awaits arousal from a dormant state. It is colourless and has no form. It is depicted by a thousand-petal lotus flower and represents the divine bliss of the couple, the seat for Shiva and Shakti.

There is a further important centre known as **Bindu**. It is a secret chakra, as it were, located on top of the head, and is the point at which the soul enters and leaves the body. In some death rituals of Nepal, a small tuft of hair is cut from the deceased person before burial or cremation.

Ayurveda and Meditation

There are two aspects of human spiritual development. There is that concerned with the body and that concerned with the mind. What are the spiritual tools of meditation that expand the mind?

We are not concerned here with the physical body, but with the subtle, and to some extent, the casual body. The tools of meditation are imaginary essences or spirits of the human body. There are a series of defined terms that represent these different layers or keys of discovery.

Agni (fire) is the symbolic fire essence, the solar flow that brings growth, expansion and transformation. It is the Shakti in Shiva, the female aspect of man. It is the hot raging energy. **Soma** (fluid) is the cooling essence; it is a lunar flow that brings creation, joy, and beauty. It is the Shiva in Shakti, the male aspect of the female, the cool lunar semen and sexual energy. An individual personality can be characterised as either *agni* or *soma*, where one aspect is dominant. He or she might be a fire or water person.

Agni and Soma combine for creation in Vayu, the air and wind. Vayu is the offspring of life, the prana or life energy that brings a new spiritual dimension. All three of them, Agni, Soma and Vayu, come from Surya, the sun god worshipped in some parts of India. In the Vedas, the self is said to dwell in the sun as light.

Meditation is desirable as a part of the healing process. For Ayurvedic cures to be used to their optimum, one should first bring the spiritual elements to a calm state. During meditation one turns inward. The mind is emptied of normal sensory awareness and drawn into a coma-like state, where a deep quietness is reached. The energy forces available to a mind at peace increase, and can be channelled to enhance harmony and, through that, healing. In meditation one seeks to find pure consciousness, the focal point of un-awareness, detached from objects, reality and physical space.

The mind can exist in three conditions. These are **Manas**, **Citta** and **Buddhi**.

Manas is the ability to see the real world by using the five senses. It relates to emotion, fear etc, and is like a sixth sense. Manas helps in developing the ojas.

Citta is that which allows us to feel and know things. It is the deeper appreciation of things within the mind. It is unattached to the senses. Prana and emotion are linked to citta. The feelings, emotions, the cravings for life and rebirth connect in citta.

Buddhi is the mind of reasoning, discerning truth. It links to the discriminating mind. It is independent of the senses and is behind the power of spiritual transformation.

All three function in the subtle body and the normal body. They function between our ego and our self, or soul. Meditation is the link between these three conditions of the mind and the three conditions of the body. Yoga is the exercise that stimulates these essences and the subtleties of the mind by physical or mental expansion.

There are any number of ways to meditate. The most important prerequisite is a quiet and calm environment. Meditation can be done without physical movement, or it can be done using yoga or tantra, where physical actions are performed. Imagination and visualisation are the main tools of meditation in motionless methods. By drawing in imagined light energy through the body, one can cleanse and remove undesired thoughts and forces, in order to reach a pure calmness. There are different yoga practices to provide a similar cleansing of the mind. At one extreme, the tantric sexual methods of achieving a meditative state can be used.

Chakra meditation is similar to other methods of meditation and it too relies on imagination and visualisation. In order to meditate one should sit in the lotus position — upright, with legs crossed — or lie still horizontally. Visualise light being drawn down through the different chakras to the root or base chakra, expelling negative or disturbing thoughts as you pass each point. Then imagine the chakras flowing clockwise and anti-clockwise.

One should emerge fresh and revitalised after slowly coming to conscious awareness. Breathing should be slow and controlled.

Yoga for developing prana is mainly based on methods of controlled breathing. In doing this one may find it useful, while following a breathing regime, to focus on space or the void. Space will always be filled by prana.

Ayurveda and Tantra

When we start to explore the sexual aspect of healthy living, we inevitably cross the path of Tantric ideas. What is Tantra?

The word Tantra is somewhat confusing in itself. From the Sanskrit, it means liberation, an expansion of ideas. Taken literally, it also means an expansion tool, a way of increasing the awareness of the mind to reach the divine level. Tantra is like a text called self-realisation. It is a spiritual path, an energetic route that uses rituals, meditation and mantras.

Tantric yoga seeks to expand the consciousness through exercise and physical means. An extension of this is the range of Tantric sexual rituals, in which we aim to reach a higher level of consciousness, peace of mind and enlightenment. Everything comes from the union of generative forces.

Tantra can be approached on another plane, that involving spiritual meditation. One approach is a purely meditative method, where anything and everything in the mind can be used. Through this Karmic form of Yoga one tries to consider 'thought' and abstract paths. Every action has a reaction.

The other method invokes worship of the forms of the goddess. The goddess is female wisdom. This method involves outer worship of deities through pujas, physical actions which are purely devotional. It also requires deep concentration and a clear mind to explore the inner state. It invokes the spirits of the goddesses, as forms of Shakti, to explore the relationship between our own being and the universe, the cosmos of the higher plane.

Lifestyle

The overriding principle behind Ayurveda is that every person is an individual, with his or her own constitution. Although we are all made up of the same physical constituent parts, it is clear that we do not all have identical desires and capabilities, regardless of our upbringing or education.

As discussed earlier, Ayurveda identifies our individual constitutions as Vata, Pitta or Kapha, with possible combinations of the three doshas. Just as an infinite number of colours can be mixed from the three primary colours of red, blue and yellow, so can any number of different constitutions result from different combinations of the three doshas.

But whatever our constitutional make-up, there are certain rules and recommendations for life which will help us to live free from disease, enjoying good health and happiness. Ayurveda is not only about curing disease; it is also about preventing it from happening in the first place. But it is not a religion, and does not require any belief in a supreme being. Although derived from the Hindu holy books, it has a lot in common with Buddhism, in that it recommends moderation in everything.

It is not unusual for people who begin life with a vata constitution to become kapha dominant as they get older. In fact, most of us have a tendency to put on middle age spread! In order to avoid this, it is necessary to increase our exercise levels and watch our diet.

The following routine is a recommended way of living, in keeping with the principles of Ayurveda:—

Recommended Daily Routine

Anyone who has been to India or Nepal will have seen how the streets begin to come alive at sunrise, despite the fact that businesses tend to open at the same times as in the west, i.e. 9 a.m. Before the advent of electricity, it was normal to rise and sleep with the sun, and indeed this still happens to this day in the remote mountain villages of Nepal and India. It may not be so practical to incorporate into a western lifestyle, but nevertheless some of the following points should be taken into account.

Wake before sunrise

Evacuate your bladder and bowels

Clean your teeth, tongue, hands and eyes

Sniff two drops of sesame oil into each nostril

Gargle with sesame oil

Shave and trim your nails

Take physical exercise as appropriate

Massage yourself to stimulate the body

Have a bath or shower

Dress in clean, comfortable clothing

Meditate around sunrise

Eat a light breakfast before 8 a.m.

Work or study

Midday meal, according to constitution and season
Continue work or study
Meditate again near sunset

Eat a light evening meal
Go for a short walk
Pursue light enjoyable activities
Have sexual intercourse if appropriate
Go to sleep before 10 p.m.

Diet

Ayurveda does not have one diet. The human being is a complex organism, as we have said, and "one man's meat may be another man's poison", to quote an old saying. Vitamins, calories, proteins, fat, carbohydrates and trace elements can be beneficial or detrimental depending on the circumstances. What is essential is for the energies of the diet to complement the disturbed bio-energies of the person, leading to a balanced result.

An improper diet is often the cause of an illness. Chronic illnesses often do not show any visible signs for many years, because the human organism fights against disease and unhealthy habits on its own as far as possible. Then when it can no longer do so, disease suddenly develops. This is often the case with heart attacks, cancer, diabetes and rheumatism.

Food also has an effect on our mental state and this factor is often ignored. Emotions often affect our digestion, and an upset digestive system can upset our psyche. We have earlier mentioned the three states of mind: - sattva, rajas, and tamas. These three words can also be used to categorise different types of food.

Sattva foods are light and fresh. They open the consciousness and bring harmony. So long as they are eaten in the right amount, they do not cause illness. They are fresh, juicy, oily, nutritious and sweet. For example, wheat, rice, rye, milk, butter, honey, raw sugar, green and leafy vegetables, fruit and nuts. Because they are fresh, no more than eight hours should pass in between preparing and eating these foods.

Rajas foods are passionate. They include spicy, salty, hot and dry foods such as garlic, wine, beer, tea, coffee, fizzy drinks, food fried in oil, curries and other spicy foods. These passionate foods are necessary in today's world; they stimulate ambition, motivation and sensuality, as well as fantasy, mania, jealousy and egotism. As we fight for survival in the hectic world of the twenty-first century, we need foods to give us this vital energy, but it is important not to eat too much of them – we need a balance of lighter foods as well.

Tamas foods require a lot of energy for their digestion. They increase pessimism, ignorance, greed, laziness and lack of good sense. Included in this category are canned and frozen food, leftovers, peanuts, alcoholic drinks, dried milk, root vegetables (other than sweet ones) and strong medicine. Meat falls into this group as well, despite its high nutritional value.

Other important factors are the time of day, season, frequency of eating and the atmosphere at the table. The digestive system is at its most active from 10 a.m. till 2 p.m., and this is the best time for eating the main meal. A pleasant atmosphere at the dining table helps digestion; no arguments and no talking or laughing while eating.

Eating between meals is not recommended, except when carrying out hard physical work, and then only when the last meal has been properly digested.

It is not always the case that a diet is based on the person's bio-type alone. Age and gender must also be taken into account. Older people should eat an anti-vata diet, those of middle age should eat an anti-pitta diet, and a child's diet should be anti-kapha.

How is it possible to cook for all the family at the same time? It may seem difficult to comprehend, based on all the previous information we have discussed. But in fact families tend to be of the same type or close; bio-type is influenced by heredity. And the same food can be prepared hot or cold, with or without spices, cooked or raw.

Ayurveda in Modern Times

With all the developments of the modern world, we may well ask, why Ayurveda? Nowadays more and more people are turning to the ancient philosophies, to seek to live in harmony with themselves and the world, to avoid filling their bodies with unnecessary chemicals. Western medicine has progressed so far, with drugs producing miraculous cures, but often with unwanted side effects. Pollution and food additives create their own problems; we are in many ways killing and injuring ourselves.

But why should we go back thousands of years to find the answer to healthy living? Some of the concepts of Ayurveda are indeed difficult to comprehend to a Westerner used to living in a scientific world where everything has to have a proof. Why should we believe all this "airy-fairy nonsense" about physically non-existent channels and doshas etc? Perhaps because so many people with chronic diseases have been failed by Western medicine, turned away because their disease does not fit any classic pattern, but Ayurveda has found a solution for them.

Our bodies are immensely complex organisms, to which no one knows all the answers, so is it not therefore possible that the ancient masters of so long ago still have something to teach us, something that was perhaps more clear in the less complicated world of the Vedas?

"All truths are easy to understand
once they are discovered.
The point is to discover them"

— Galileo Galilei

Bibliography

AYURVEDA The Science of Self-Healing Dr Vasant Lad; Motilal Banarsidass Publishers Pvt. Ltd.

THE HANDBOOK OF AYURVEDA Dr Shantha Godagama; Kyle Cathie Ltd.

For more details about Pilgrims
and other books published by them
you may visit our website at
www.pilgrimsbooks.com
or
for Mail Order and Catalogue
contact us at

Sanjay

MORE TITLES ON HEALTH FROM PILGRIMS PUBLISHING